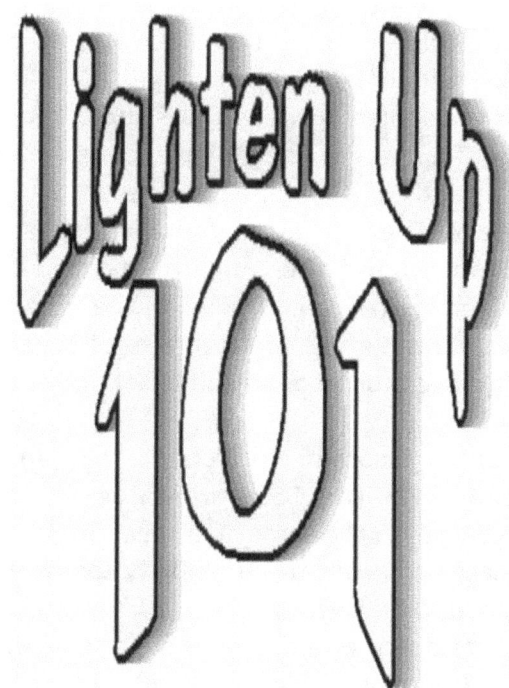

101
"Weighs"
To Laugh
Away The Pounds

By Rich DiGirolamo & Michelle Gotay

So here's the story:

I am overweight. I met Rich. He *used* to be overweight. He told me that I didn't *have* to be overweight anymore. I told him to jump in a lake.

I guess the subject of weight loss and dieting is a bit of a sore spot for me. You see, I have lost and gained hundreds of pounds in my life, each time a greater struggle than the last. The thought of embarking on another torturous journey down the weight-(hate) loss trail leaves me less than motivated. I have in the past associated weight loss and dieting with feelings of dread, deprivation, guilt, obsession and difficulty (not unlike my former marriage...).

Apparently, according to Rich, there *is* another way. "FUN" and "WEIGHT-LOSS" are three words I would have NEVER put in the same sentence, but Rich has challenged me to consider the possibility that losing weight doesn't have to be awful.

So we sat down one day over sugar-free, fat-free vanilla lattes (thank you, Mr. Starbuck) and put together a list of ways we could (actually that **I** could) "Lighten Up" throughout this process. I know only one thing for sure... Being miserable with a bad attitude towards weight-loss has lead to short-lived successes and frown lines.

So, I told Rich that I would try it *his* way this time. I have promised to "Lighten Up", smile once in a while, and ease up on myself whenever possible. Feel free to join me in this process. Who knows? Maybe we both can laugh our way back into the jeans we have hiding in the back of our closets.

Yours in Cellulite,
Michelle

1. Attach a photo of your head to a photo of your favorite body and visualize how great you will soon be looking and feeling. Keep that visual with you at all times. Mentally rehearsing the new you will help achieve success.

2. Record yourself chewing carrot sticks and celery. Play the tape as background "music" at your next dinner party; while your guests are pigging out. Tell your friends it is your new weight loss sound machine.

3. Take photos of yourself wearing the same clothes at different points in your weight loss journey. Place pictures next to each other and identify/circle differences in the photos.

4. Make a paper doll of yourself and cut out clothing from a magazine or catalogue that you love. Dress yourself up in the way you want to look. Do not be afraid to be a bit risqué.

5. Design a pin that says, "Congratulate me. I'm a LOSER." Celebrating your success keeps you constantly involved in your process.

6. Make up your own theme song to sing or hum while you work out. (e.g. theme from "STOCKY"). Change the words as you go through your weight loss process.

7. Create a "Skinny Dip" jar. Every time you treat yourself well by eating right or exercising (even when you didn't feel like it), put money ($1.00?) into this fund. Periodically "dip" into the jar and get yourself something you deserve (preferably not a dinner).

8. Draw a big graph to hang on your refrigerator monitoring your weight loss. No need to put numbers on it for all to see (unless you choose to). You know where you started. Make the graph in one or two pound increments. Buy some colored markers to

document your weekly progress. Smaller increments will appear as greater losses.

9. Be sure to take "before" and "after" shots. Monitoring your success is key to future success. (I know you don't want to take the "before" shots, but you will be glad you did later.

10. Design post cards to send to your friends and family (those who *are* supportive) announcing the return of your true self.

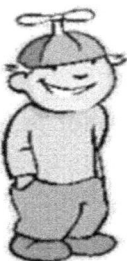

Are you skinny yet? I'm heading to my mailbox. Send a note to:

PO Box 584
Marion CT 06444, USA

11. Write "Dear John" letters to your favorite, less healthy foods. Explain that you miss them, but you have moved on and cannot be with them in the same way you were before. Be gentle; they have feelings too.

12. Throw a farewell party to the part of yourself that keeps you down. Invite only your closest friends. Say goodbye to your old self, thank him or her for what he/she taught you, and dance the night away.

13. Connect with others who are losing weight and have a recipe contest. Only healthy, delicious foods need be entered. Ask a thin person and a not-so-thin person to be the judges. You want a panel of judges who are not biased. The winner gets thinner.

14. Buy a punching bag. Tape a picture or package wrapper of that food which is your toughest enemy to the bag. Get in the "ring" when you're feeling a binge come on. Beat the bag for a few rounds, and before you know it, the crisis will be over. As you are punching, be sure you tell that wrapper how difficult they are making your life. Works well with pictures of spouses too.

15. Celebrate a tempting moment. Make up a cheer that you (or others) can do for yourself when you use particular restraint in a difficult situation.   Pom-poms are optional. (Example: "2-4-6-8 Debbie didn't eat the cake! Yeeeea...Debbie!")

16. Put a cocktail umbrella in your lemon water. It might make you feel happier. If possible, arrange to have your lemon water served to you by a gorgeous babe/hunk on a tropical island.

17. Take your exercise to new places. Jog at the mall (just don't be carrying a purse) or climb the stairs at fancy hotels. Get to know the doormen.

18. Make a list of all the people who made fun of your excess weight and send them a thank you for their nasty motivational techniques. Be sure to include a picture of you in your new bikini.

19. Cut up your charge card from the "plus size store". Mail it back to the store with a letter telling them you will no longer be needing their services. Thank them for being there when you needed them most.

20. Take pledges for pounds lost. Create your own for-profit organization- F. A. T. "Free And Thin". While they're feeling sorry for you, you are buying new

clothes with their money!

21. Start up a pool with your coworkers regarding the date you reach your weight loss goal, number of times you gain weight back before you do, and number of times you hit a coworker out of frustration and hunger. Split the pot with the winner

22. Create a "Calorie Gallery". Purchase large quantities of clay to create sculptures. The weight of the sculpture should reflect your weight lost to date.

23. Stand naked in front of the mirror. Try not to laugh.

To answer your question, Rich......No.
I am NOT skinny, but the mirror and I are *both* having a good chuckle!

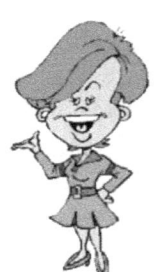

24. Stand naked in front of the mirror. See if you can identify shapes or familiar characters in your fat rolls (kind of like you do when looking at cloud formations).

25. Place an ad in your local newspaper. LOST- # pounds. If found, please do NOT return to (your name), (your address).

26. Place an ad in your local newspaper. LOST- # pounds. If found, please deliver to (name of your enemy), (enemy's address).

27. Find ways to use your hidden junk food and turn it into modern art. Give the masterpieces as holiday gifts.

28. Post WANTED posters of yourself at the local convenience store, bakery or deli (or wherever it is you get your binging goods) so that you'll be less likely to enter:

WANTED FOR SELF-ABUSE
(your name and photograph here)
May be considered big-armed and dangerous (to his/her own health)
If spotted, immediately hug and call authorities
(someone who's been there)

29. Drink all highly caloric beverages only from a dribble glass. (Avoid grape juice) Or be responsible and use the smallest glass you can find.

30. Take up belly dancing. Chances are, your belly could use the workout, and as it diminishes, your self-esteem may enlarge.

31. Build your confidence. Tell people that you already/always knew you had a pretty face....Now they should check out the rest of you.

> Well, it looks like your boobs and feet are shrinking... Good for you!

32. Walk down supermarket aisles. Have conversations with people about their poor food choices. If you are bashful, just smile to yourself.

33. Have target practice with leftover picnic/BBQ food. This is a great way to have guests help with clean-up.

34. Act like a kid. Have a food fight with leftovers. Hope-fully you are now a smaller target.

35. Throw a party on April Fool's Day. Fill your keg with diet cream soda. Act drunk.

36. Instead of "Just Married", write your weight loss on your rear car window. Update losses regularly. I.e. "Just Lost 10 lbs!"

37. Introduce yourself to strangers as "Ilene Now".

38. Rent a billboard. Display your fat picture asking "Have you seen this person? Well you should see her now!"

39. Host a party without food. Show others that food does not have to be the center of all activities. It really doesn't. Watch guests reactions. Play party games. See who is the first to leave.

40. Design an easy exercise plan. Set your clock a few minutes late each morning; forcing yourself to run to the train, bus or plane. Set the clock later and later as you improve.

41. Post "No Fatty, Greasy, and Fried Foods Allowed on Premises" signs in your kitchen.

42. Have a personalized doormat made. Some ideas might be Beware of Dieter or Bitchy Dieter Lives Here. This will let people know you are serious about your health and weight loss efforts this time and fore-warn them of possible violent mood swings.

43. Carry a pocket mirror with you. Hold it up to the fac-es of people offering unsolicited weight loss advice.

44. When someone noticing your weight loss asks, "are you sick?" , reply "Yes, I'm dying" You must be able to hold a straight face for this one.

45. Commission an artist to paint/draw your portrait at your desired weight. Hang it proudly. Airbrush appropriate trouble spots.

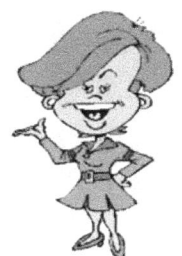

"Possible violent mood swings"?! I can go from happy to sad in 3.2 seconds!

46. Reward yourself with that piece of jewelry/trip/automobile/new home you have been wanting when you reach a significant point in your weight loss journey.

47. Host a pageant show for yourself. Invite only those bigger than you. Wear all of those outfits in your closet that still have the tags on them. Share the story behind the outfit (i.e. "I was supposed to wear this the summer of 1963")

48. Your mother told you to share. So, offer your "fat" clothes to your larger-than-you friends and family. Do it lovingly, of course.

49. Buy an obnoxiously short pair of running shorts, a tank top and an afro wig and make your own exercise video. (Oh wait...that has been done, but yours will be better.)

50. Introduce yourself as follows (all the time) "hi, my name is _____. I've lost _____ pounds". Positive affirmation breeds success.

51. Create the world's biggest salad. At the time of this printing there was too much conflicting information, but it will have to be at least 2,212 square kilometers in size. Invite a small country to share it with you.

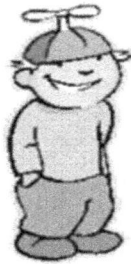

"Hi, I'm Rich...I've lost my patience with... Michelle!"

52. Host a "Thinner Dinner" and serve the absolute worst diet food you can find. Watch reactions. Cardboard-like crackers (you know the ones) with lettuce and mustard, followed by broth and grapefruit.

53. Buy some cable TV time. Do a commercial on how to lose weight. Please share some of the ideas in this booklet – along with the authors' names.

54. Cable advertising is cheap. Run a cable TV advertise-ment sharing your weight loss.

55. Enlist your friends in your weight loss endeavor. Host a low fat dinner party fundraiser. Charge $100 per head. Donate all profits to a local soup kitchen.

56. Your large clothes have many uses. Host an art exhibit of things you can do with large underwear. Please remove stains first.

57. Make a list of all of the faults of those people who comment on your weight. Post it (anonymously) in local hot spots.

58. This one might require some venture capital. Start your own designer apparel line. The largest size will be an 8.

59. Burn all your "fat" clothes. For those of you with a significant weight loss, you may wish to contact your local fire department first.

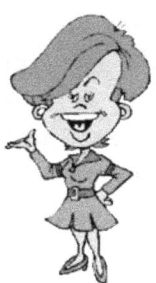

It seems my work-out clothes are flame-resistant. Could this be a sign?

60. Hire a skywriter to announce you've reached your goal weight. It is now safe for you to ride in the plane yourself.

61. Lust is a great source of motivation. Hang a naked picture of someone you lust after directly across from you while eating dinner.

62. Eat your meals naked. You will recognize success when you find you are able to do this with another.

63. Learn to eat slower. If necessary, use a slotted spoon or chopsticks. Proficient chopstickers should try using only one chopstick.

64. Have as much sex as possible to help the pounds come off. As the pounds come off, so does the blind-fold....as the weight goes down, the lights can come up.

65. Throw healthy foods into the shopping carts of over-weight people. Don't worry about being able to run away from them. Remember, they are overweight.

66. Sleep with the spouse/partner/significant other of the "evil one" who makes fun of you. Please remember that the purpose of this booklet is to have some fun along with generating many useful ideas. But if he/she is cute....

67. Invite the "Skinny Twit's" kids over to have lunch with your kids. Feed his/her children fattening foods. When the sugar high is at its maximum, send them home.

68. Organize a "Run for the K.A.K.E." event in your town. When you figure out what K.AK.E. stands for let us know. We forgot.

69. For each pound you have shed, store a pound of lard in your refrigerator. If it becomes necessary to pur-chase a commercial size refrigerator, assume you have succeeded.

70. Recalibrate the scale before your significant other gets on.

71. Reward yourself Certificates of Success. Earn enough to wallpaper your largest room.

72. Float in a diet root beer bath. Do not forget the straws and that your mother taught you to share.

73. Write your own version of "the Battle of the Bulge".

74. Find/make new friends....ones that actually under-stand.

75. Stop giving people advice on how to lose weight and start following it. Yes. Ouch! That hurt some of you. Too bad.

Be gentle when they (for once) ask you, "Do I look fat?"

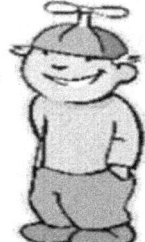

76. Buy an outfit in the size you want to be. Try it on regularly. Please be realistic. You were a size two at birth.

77. What is that one thing you have secretly desired to wear? Fishnets? Leather pants? A thong? Buy it. Prepare to wear it. Try it on at regular intervals. Please do not suffocate.

78. Have a burning. Buy one of those outdoor decorative chimneys and burn all the foods that have caused you grief. Do not burn yourself trying to save any of your old friends.

79. Have another burning. Burn pictures of all of those people who would not give you the right time of day when you were overweight.

80. Lose weight with a friend. Find a friend who is trying to lose weight as well; eat meals together on a regular basis.

81. Play with produce. I know what you are thinking… shame on you. Go to the supermarket and pick up a piece of produce you have never eaten. Buy it and

plan an entire meal around that piece of produce. Yes, this may require some research.

> Oh.....it turns out that caramel apples are NOT produce... I think I'm getting the hang of this...

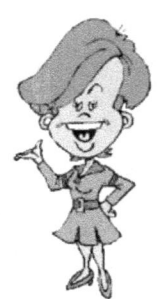

82. As you start losing weight donate your big clothes to a shelter or some other charity. Feel proud that someone is benefiting from your loss.

83. Donate a certain amount of money per pound lost to a favorite charity. Please tell them the story behind your donation. Encourage their involvement to support you.

84. Decorate your walls with pictures of those Skinny people you want to emulate. C'mon you did it when you were a kid with posters of teen heart throbs.

85. Reward yourself for each five pounds lost. Take in a movie. Get a massage. Buy a new tune.

86. Do the hustle. Buy some of your favorite music from an era of your youth. Dance on a regular basis. Dancing leads to weight loss and cardiovascular strength.

87. Host parties to celebrate your weight loss. Perhaps celebrate each size lower. Prepare the low fat and low calorie meals that got you to this next level. Play games. Wear your best new outfit.

88. Come out. Announce your weight loss through email, letters or postcards. Let everyone know how much hotter you are getting.

89. Buy a carnival mirror. You know the one; the one that makes you look long and lank. Watch yourself shrink. Use until a standard mirror is tolerable or appropriate.

90. Sell your weight on Ebay. It's just a few pennies but I am sure you will get a bid or two. It should at least get you an email or two. And hey, who knows maybe a date.

91. Prepare a YouTube video of your weight loss. Include pictures and videos of when you started and points along the "weigh". Don't forget the video clips of you exercising.

> Are you skinny YET? I'm still waiting to hear from you. Too cheap to buy a stamp? Email me: rich@richdigirolamo.com

92. Put labels on foods that might cause you to overeat. Label them as "Poison" or "Crap" or "Urine". Feed them to your loved ones when they aggravate you.

93. Eat wearing sexy lingerie. We mean food.

94. Try a week of healthy ethnic eating. Chinese, Japanese and even Italian can all be healthy when done right. Try seven different ethnic cuisines in one week.

95. Set up a shrine in your home where you can pray that certain people in your life get bigger. Include pictures of those people. Pray to the God/Goddess of Fat.

96. Exercise for free. Join every gym in your area that offers a free two-week membership. Make sure you quit before the two weeks are up. Do not join gyms simultaneously. Do not tell them where you received this tip.

97. Hang around with people larger than you. It is great for the ego. It also gives you the opportunity to be the weight loss poster child. Buy a copy of this book for each of those people. You can afford it. You are eating less.

98. Enlist a good friend to act as your "pantry monitor". Give this person permission to, periodically and without warning, put your home back in "SAFE MODE".

99. Use your cookie cutters to make interesting meat and vegetable shapes. Do this especially at holiday time so as not to feel a loss. Did you ever try a snowman potato slice?

100. Seek out fellow "fatties" at the next party you attend. Stick together and help to see each other through the dessert buffet.

101. Host your own Lighten Up 101 evening of fun. Buy LOTS and LOTS of these books for all attendees. Read through the book together. Laugh, share your thoughts and crazy ideas regarding these 101 tips. The object is to spark new ideas that lead you down your personal road to weight loss success. Always remember, the more you laugh, the more calories ou burn. Have fun.

Special Tip #102: Always remember where you came from. Once you become skinny, please do not become one of the unsupportive people referred to in the book.

Hey Rich, did you get my picture postcard _YET?!_

I've been thinking... maybe we should take this show on the road!

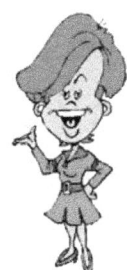

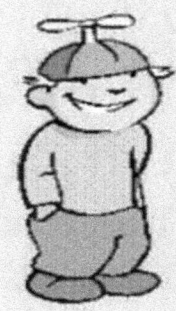

Imagine splitting your pants and running around New York City looking for a needle and thread at 7:00AM; only to end up using a stapler to repair the damage. Don't laugh!

For years I dieted the way most people diet – with the short term in mind. I made it a painful, boring, and depriving experience. I did the yo-yo thing. Can you relate? Then one day I decided to get serious - or should I say have some serious fun losing weight.

Fast forward…… Thirty-two pounds are gone. Then this blast of red hair comes into my life – we will call her Tushelle for these purposes. All she did was whine about being fat and how it was impossible to lose weight and keep it off. After restraining myself to not back my car into her, I asked her what was really eating her? Ouch! Yes, that one hurt!

After we removed the dagger from my heart we let the games begin. I shared with Tushelle how I learned to make weight-loss fun, and all the fun I have experienced years later not dragging around that excess baggage – and so could she.

For information regarding quantity purchases of this book, personal development workshops, coaching or other speaking services contact Rich:

http://richdigirolamo.com